AF875737

Weekly Pain Log

WEEK OF ____________

0	1	2	3	4	5	6	7	8	9	10

LOW THREAT	GUARDED	ELEVATED	HIGH ALERT	SEVERE
LIFE IS RICH	NO LOUD, CROWDED, FAR PLACES	DRAGGING/ LAGGING	EDGY, DEEP, DULL, ACHY	PULSING, THROBBING, SHOOTING, STABBING, BURNING

Date	Time	Color Scale Number	Symptom Area	Precipitating Event	Coping Strategy	Meds	Results

Weekly Pain Log

WEEK OF ____________

0 1	2 3	4 5	6 7	8 9 10
LOW THREAT	GUARDED	ELEVATED	HIGH ALERT	SEVERE
LIFE IS RICH	NO LOUD, CROWDED, FAR PLACES	DRAGGING/ LAGGING	EDGY, DEEP, DULL, ACHY	PULSING, THROBBING, SHOOTING, STABBING, BURNING

Date	Time	Color Scale Number	Symptom Area	Precipitating Event	Coping Strategy	Meds	Results

Weekly Pain Log

WEEK OF ____________

0 1	2 3	4 5	6 7	8 9 10
LOW THREAT	GUARDED	ELEVATED	HIGH ALERT	SEVERE
LIFE IS RICH	NO LOUD, CROWDED, FAR PLACES	DRAGGING/ LAGGING	EDGY, DEEP, DULL, ACHY	PULSING, THROBBING, SHOOTING, STABBING, BURNING

Date	Time	Color Scale Number	Symptom Area	Precipitating Event	Coping Strategy	Meds	Results

Weekly Pain Log

WEEK OF ____________________

0	1	2	3	4	5	6	7	8	9	10
LOW THREAT		GUARDED		ELEVATED		HIGH ALERT		SEVERE		
LIFE IS RICH		NO LOUD, CROWDED, FAR PLACES		DRAGGING/ LAGGING		EDGY, DEEP, DULL, ACHY		PULSING, THROBBING, SHOOTING, STABBING, BURNING		

Date	Time	Color Scale Number	Symptom Area	Precipitating Event	Coping Strategy	Meds	Results

Weekly Pain Log

WEEK OF ______________

0 1	2 3	4 5	6 7	8 9 10
LOW THREAT	GUARDED	ELEVATED	HIGH ALERT	SEVERE
LIFE IS RICH	NO LOUD, CROWDED, FAR PLACES	DRAGGING/ LAGGING	EDGY, DEEP, DULL, ACHY	PULSING, THROBBING, SHOOTING, STABBING, BURNING

Date	Time	Color Scale Number	Symptom Area	Precipitating Event	Coping Strategy	Meds	Results

Weekly Pain Log

WEEK OF ______________________

0 1	2 3	4 5	6 7	8 9 10
LOW THREAT	GUARDED	ELEVATED	HIGH ALERT	SEVERE
LIFE IS RICH	NO LOUD, CROWDED, FAR PLACES	DRAGGING/ LAGGING	EDGY, DEEP, DULL, ACHY	PULSING, THROBBING, SHOOTING, STABBING, BURNING

Date	Time	Color Scale Number	Symptom Area	Precipitating Event	Coping Strategy	Meds	Results

Weekly Pain Log

WEEK OF ____________

0 1	2 3	4 5	6 7	8 9 10
LOW THREAT	GUARDED	ELEVATED	HIGH ALERT	SEVERE
LIFE IS RICH	NO LOUD, CROWDED, FAR PLACES	DRAGGING/ LAGGING	EDGY, DEEP, DULL, ACHY	PULSING, THROBBING, SHOOTING, STABBING, BURNING

Date	Time	Color Scale Number	Symptom Area	Precipitating Event	Coping Strategy	Meds	Results

Weekly Pain Log

WEEK OF ____________________

0 1	2 3	4 5	6 7	8 9 10
LOW THREAT	**GUARDED**	**ELEVATED**	**HIGH ALERT**	**SEVERE**
LIFE IS RICH	NO LOUD, CROWDED, FAR PLACES	DRAGGING/ LAGGING	EDGY, DEEP, DULL, ACHY	PULSING, THROBBING, SHOOTING, STABBING, BURNING

Date	Time	Color Scale Number	Symptom Area	Precipitating Event	Coping Strategy	Meds	Results

Weekly Pain Log

WEEK OF ____________

0 – 1	2 – 3	4 – 5	6 – 7	8 – 9 – 10
LOW THREAT	GUARDED	ELEVATED	HIGH ALERT	SEVERE
LIFE IS RICH	NO LOUD, CROWDED, FAR PLACES	DRAGGING/ LAGGING	EDGY, DEEP, DULL, ACHY	PULSING, THROBBING, SHOOTING, STABBING, BURNING

Date	Time	Color Scale Number	Symptom Area	Precipitating Event	Coping Strategy	Meds	Results

Weekly Pain Log

WEEK OF ____________________

0	1	2	3	4	5	6	7	8	9	10
LOW THREAT		GUARDED		ELEVATED		HIGH ALERT		SEVERE		
LIFE IS RICH		NO LOUD, CROWDED, FAR PLACES		DRAGGING/ LAGGING		EDGY, DEEP, DULL, ACHY		PULSING, THROBBING, SHOOTING, STABBING, BURNING		

Date	Time	Color Scale Number	Symptom Area	Precipitating Event	Coping Strategy	Meds	Results

Weekly Pain Log

WEEK OF ____________________

0 1	2 3	4 5	6 7	8 9 10
LOW THREAT	GUARDED	ELEVATED	HIGH ALERT	SEVERE
LIFE IS RICH	NO LOUD, CROWDED, FAR PLACES	DRAGGING/ LAGGING	EDGY, DEEP, DULL, ACHY	PULSING, THROBBING, SHOOTING, STABBING, BURNING

Date	Time	Color Scale Number	Symptom Area	Precipitating Event	Coping Strategy	Meds	Results

Weekly Pain Log

WEEK OF ____________________

0	1	2	3	4	5	6	7	8	9	10
LOW THREAT		GUARDED		ELEVATED		HIGH ALERT		SEVERE		
LIFE IS RICH		NO LOUD, CROWDED, FAR PLACES		DRAGGING/ LAGGING		EDGY, DEEP, DULL, ACHY		PULSING, THROBBING, SHOOTING, STABBING, BURNING		

Date	Time	Color Scale Number	Symptom Area	Precipitating Event	Coping Strategy	Meds	Results

Weekly Pain Log

WEEK OF ____________

0	1	2	3	4	5	6	7	8	9	10
LOW THREAT		GUARDED		ELEVATED		HIGH ALERT		SEVERE		
LIFE IS RICH		NO LOUD, CROWDED, FAR PLACES		DRAGGING/ LAGGING		EDGY, DEEP, DULL, ACHY		PULSING, THROBBING, SHOOTING, STABBING, BURNING		

Date	Time	Color Scale Number	Symptom Area	Precipitating Event	Coping Strategy	Meds	Results

Weekly Pain Log

WEEK OF ____________________

0 1	2 3	4 5	6 7	8 9 10
LOW THREAT	GUARDED	ELEVATED	HIGH ALERT	SEVERE
LIFE IS RICH	NO LOUD, CROWDED, FAR PLACES	DRAGGING/ LAGGING	EDGY, DEEP, DULL, ACHY	PULSING, THROBBING, SHOOTING, STABBING, BURNING

Date	Time	Color Scale Number	Symptom Area	Precipitating Event	Coping Strategy	Meds	Results

Weekly Pain Log

WEEK OF ______________

0	1	2	3	4	5	6	7	8	9	10
LOW THREAT		GUARDED		ELEVATED		HIGH ALERT		SEVERE		
LIFE IS RICH		NO LOUD, CROWDED, FAR PLACES		DRAGGING/ LAGGING		EDGY, DEEP, DULL, ACHY		PULSING, THROBBING, SHOOTING, STABBING, BURNING		

Date	Time	Color Scale Number	Symptom Area	Precipitating Event	Coping Strategy	Meds	Results

Weekly Pain Log

WEEK OF ____________________

0 1	2 3	4 5	6 7	8 9 10
LOW THREAT	GUARDED	ELEVATED	HIGH ALERT	SEVERE
LIFE IS RICH	NO LOUD, CROWDED, FAR PLACES	DRAGGING/ LAGGING	EDGY, DEEP, DULL, ACHY	PULSING, THROBBING, SHOOTING, STABBING, BURNING

Date	Time	Color Scale Number	Symptom Area	Precipitating Event	Coping Strategy	Meds	Results

Weekly Pain Log

WEEK OF ____________

0	1	2	3	4	5	6	7	8	9	10
LOW THREAT		GUARDED		ELEVATED		HIGH ALERT		SEVERE		
LIFE IS RICH		NO LOUD, CROWDED, FAR PLACES		DRAGGING/ LAGGING		EDGY, DEEP, DULL, ACHY		PULSING, THROBBING, SHOOTING, STABBING, BURNING		

Date	Time	Color Scale Number	Symptom Area	Precipitating Event	Coping Strategy	Meds	Results

Weekly Pain Log

WEEK OF ____________________

0 1	2 3	4 5	6 7	8 9 10
LOW THREAT	GUARDED	ELEVATED	HIGH ALERT	SEVERE
LIFE IS RICH	NO LOUD, CROWDED, FAR PLACES	DRAGGING/ LAGGING	EDGY, DEEP, DULL, ACHY	PULSING, THROBBING, SHOOTING, STABBING, BURNING

Date	Time	Color Scale Number	Symptom Area	Precipitating Event	Coping Strategy	Meds	Results

Weekly Pain Log

WEEK OF ____________

0	1	2	3	4	5	6	7	8	9	10
LOW THREAT		GUARDED		ELEVATED		HIGH ALERT		SEVERE		
LIFE IS RICH		NO LOUD, CROWDED, FAR PLACES		DRAGGING/ LAGGING		EDGY, DEEP, DULL, ACHY		PULSING, THROBBING, SHOOTING, STABBING, BURNING		

Date	Time	Color Scale Number	Symptom Area	Precipitating Event	Coping Strategy	Meds	Results

Weekly Pain Log

WEEK OF ____________________

0 1	2 3	4 5	6 7	8 9 10
LOW THREAT	GUARDED	ELEVATED	HIGH ALERT	SEVERE
LIFE IS RICH	NO LOUD, CROWDED, FAR PLACES	DRAGGING/ LAGGING	EDGY, DEEP, DULL, ACHY	PULSING, THROBBING, SHOOTING, STABBING, BURNING

Date	Time	Color Scale Number	Symptom Area	Precipitating Event	Coping Strategy	Meds	Results

Weekly Pain Log

WEEK OF ____________________

0 1	2 3	4 5	6 7	8 9 10
LOW THREAT	GUARDED	ELEVATED	HIGH ALERT	SEVERE
LIFE IS RICH	NO LOUD, CROWDED, FAR PLACES	DRAGGING/ LAGGING	EDGY, DEEP, DULL, ACHY	PULSING, THROBBING, SHOOTING, STABBING, BURNING

Date	Time	Color Scale Number	Symptom Area	Precipitating Event	Coping Strategy	Meds	Results

Weekly Pain Log

WEEK OF ____________________

0	1	2	3	4	5	6	7	8	9	10
LOW THREAT		GUARDED		ELEVATED		HIGH ALERT		SEVERE		
LIFE IS RICH		NO LOUD, CROWDED, FAR PLACES		DRAGGING/ LAGGING		EDGY, DEEP, DULL, ACHY		PULSING, THROBBING, SHOOTING, STABBING, BURNING		

Date	Time	Color Scale Number	Symptom Area	Precipitating Event	Coping Strategy	Meds	Results

Weekly Pain Log

WEEK OF ______________

0	1	2	3	4	5	6	7	8	9	10
LOW THREAT		GUARDED		ELEVATED		HIGH ALERT		SEVERE		
LIFE IS RICH		NO LOUD, CROWDED, FAR PLACES		DRAGGING/ LAGGING		EDGY, DEEP, DULL, ACHY		PULSING, THROBBING, SHOOTING, STABBING, BURNING		

Date	Time	Color Scale Number	Symptom Area	Precipitating Event	Coping Strategy	Meds	Results

Weekly Pain Log

WEEK OF ____________________

0	1	2	3	4	5	6	7	8	9	10
LOW THREAT		GUARDED		ELEVATED		HIGH ALERT		SEVERE		
LIFE IS RICH		NO LOUD, CROWDED, FAR PLACES		DRAGGING/ LAGGING		EDGY, DEEP, DULL, ACHY		PULSING, THROBBING, SHOOTING, STABBING, BURNING		

Date	Time	Color Scale Number	Symptom Area	Precipitating Event	Coping Strategy	Meds	Results

Weekly Pain Log

WEEK OF ____________

0	1	2	3	4	5	6	7	8	9	10
LOW THREAT		GUARDED		ELEVATED		HIGH ALERT		SEVERE		
LIFE IS RICH		NO LOUD, CROWDED, FAR PLACES		DRAGGING/ LAGGING		EDGY, DEEP, DULL, ACHY		PULSING, THROBBING, SHOOTING, STABBING, BURNING		

Date	Time	Color Scale Number	Symptom Area	Precipitating Event	Coping Strategy	Meds	Results

Weekly Pain Log

WEEK OF ____________

0	1	2	3	4	5	6	7	8	9	10
LOW THREAT		GUARDED		ELEVATED		HIGH ALERT		SEVERE		
LIFE IS RICH		NO LOUD, CROWDED, FAR PLACES		DRAGGING/ LAGGING		EDGY, DEEP, DULL, ACHY		PULSING, THROBBING, SHOOTING, STABBING, BURNING		

Date	Time	Color Scale Number	Symptom Area	Precipitating Event	Coping Strategy	Meds	Results

Weekly Pain Log

WEEK OF ____________

0	1	2	3	4	5	6	7	8	9	10

LOW THREAT	GUARDED	ELEVATED	HIGH ALERT	SEVERE
LIFE IS RICH	NO LOUD, CROWDED, FAR PLACES	DRAGGING/ LAGGING	EDGY, DEEP, DULL, ACHY	PULSING, THROBBING, SHOOTING, STABBING, BURNING

Date	Time	Color Scale Number	Symptom Area	Precipitating Event	Coping Strategy	Meds	Results

Weekly Pain Log

WEEK OF ______________

0	1	2	3	4	5	6	7	8	9	10
LOW THREAT		GUARDED		ELEVATED		HIGH ALERT		SEVERE		
LIFE IS RICH		NO LOUD, CROWDED, FAR PLACES		DRAGGING/ LAGGING		EDGY, DEEP, DULL, ACHY		PULSING, THROBBING, SHOOTING, STABBING, BURNING		

Date	Time	Color Scale Number	Symptom Area	Precipitating Event	Coping Strategy	Meds	Results

Weekly Pain Log

WEEK OF ____________

0	1	2	3	4	5	6	7	8	9	10
LOW THREAT		GUARDED		ELEVATED		HIGH ALERT		SEVERE		
LIFE IS RICH		NO LOUD, CROWDED, FAR PLACES		DRAGGING/ LAGGING		EDGY, DEEP, DULL, ACHY		PULSING, THROBBING, SHOOTING, STABBING, BURNING		

Date	Time	Color Scale Number	Symptom Area	Precipitating Event	Coping Strategy	Meds	Results

Weekly Pain Log

WEEK OF ____________

0	1	2	3	4	5	6	7	8	9	10
LOW THREAT		GUARDED		ELEVATED		HIGH ALERT		SEVERE		
LIFE IS RICH		NO LOUD, CROWDED, FAR PLACES		DRAGGING/ LAGGING		EDGY, DEEP, DULL, ACHY		PULSING, THROBBING, SHOOTING, STABBING, BURNING		

Date	Time	Color Scale Number	Symptom Area	Precipitating Event	Coping Strategy	Meds	Results

Weekly Pain Log

WEEK OF ____________

0 1	2 3	4 5	6 7	8 9 10
LOW THREAT	GUARDED	ELEVATED	HIGH ALERT	SEVERE
LIFE IS RICH	NO LOUD, CROWDED, FAR PLACES	DRAGGING/ LAGGING	EDGY, DEEP, DULL, ACHY	PULSING, THROBBING, SHOOTING, STABBING, BURNING

Date	Time	Color Scale Number	Symptom Area	Precipitating Event	Coping Strategy	Meds	Results

Weekly Pain Log

WEEK OF ____________

0 – 1	2 – 3	4 – 5	6 – 7	8 – 9 – 10
LOW THREAT	**GUARDED**	**ELEVATED**	**HIGH ALERT**	**SEVERE**
LIFE IS RICH	NO LOUD, CROWDED, FAR PLACES	DRAGGING/ LAGGING	EDGY, DEEP, DULL, ACHY	PULSING, THROBBING, SHOOTING, STABBING, BURNING

Date	Time	Color Scale Number	Symptom Area	Precipitating Event	Coping Strategy	Meds	Results

Weekly Pain Log

WEEK OF ____________________

0 1	2 3	4 5	6 7	8 9 10
LOW THREAT	GUARDED	ELEVATED	HIGH ALERT	SEVERE
LIFE IS RICH	NO LOUD, CROWDED, FAR PLACES	DRAGGING/ LAGGING	EDGY, DEEP, DULL, ACHY	PULSING, THROBBING, SHOOTING, STABBING, BURNING

Date	Time	Color Scale Number	Symptom Area	Precipitating Event	Coping Strategy	Meds	Results

Weekly Pain Log

WEEK OF ____________________

0	1	2	3	4	5	6	7	8	9	10
LOW THREAT		GUARDED		ELEVATED		HIGH ALERT		SEVERE		
LIFE IS RICH		NO LOUD, CROWDED, FAR PLACES		DRAGGING/ LAGGING		EDGY, DEEP, DULL, ACHY		PULSING, THROBBING, SHOOTING, STABBING, BURNING		

Date	Time	Color Scale Number	Symptom Area	Precipitating Event	Coping Strategy	Meds	Results

Weekly Pain Log

WEEK OF ____________

0 1	2 3	4 5	6 7	8 9 10
LOW THREAT	GUARDED	ELEVATED	HIGH ALERT	SEVERE
LIFE IS RICH	NO LOUD, CROWDED, FAR PLACES	DRAGGING/ LAGGING	EDGY, DEEP, DULL, ACHY	PULSING, THROBBING, SHOOTING, STABBING, BURNING

Date	Time	Color Scale Number	Symptom Area	Precipitating Event	Coping Strategy	Meds	Results

Weekly Pain Log

WEEK OF ____________

0 – 1	2 – 3	4 – 5	6 – 7	8 – 9 – 10
LOW THREAT	GUARDED	ELEVATED	HIGH ALERT	SEVERE
LIFE IS RICH	NO LOUD, CROWDED, FAR PLACES	DRAGGING/ LAGGING	EDGY, DEEP, DULL, ACHY	PULSING, THROBBING, SHOOTING, STABBING, BURNING

Date	Time	Color Scale Number	Symptom Area	Precipitating Event	Coping Strategy	Meds	Results

Weekly Pain Log

VEEK OF ______________

0	1	2	3	4	5	6	7	8	9	10
LOW THREAT		GUARDED		ELEVATED		HIGH ALERT		SEVERE		
LIFE IS RICH		NO LOUD, CROWDED, FAR PLACES		DRAGGING/ LAGGING		EDGY, DEEP, DULL, ACHY		PULSING, THROBBING, SHOOTING, STABBING, BURNING		

Date	Time	Color Scale Number	Symptom Area	Precipitating Event	Coping Strategy	Meds	Results

Weekly Pain Log

WEEK OF ______________________

0 1	2 3	4 5	6 7	8 9 10
LOW THREAT	**GUARDED**	**ELEVATED**	**HIGH ALERT**	**SEVERE**
LIFE IS RICH	NO LOUD, CROWDED, FAR PLACES	DRAGGING/ LAGGING	EDGY, DEEP, DULL, ACHY	PULSING, THROBBING, SHOOTING, STABBING, BURNING

Date	Time	Color Scale Number	Symptom Area	Precipitating Event	Coping Strategy	Meds	Results

Weekly Pain Log

WEEK OF ______________

0	1	2	3	4	5	6	7	8	9	10
LOW THREAT		GUARDED		ELEVATED		HIGH ALERT		SEVERE		
LIFE IS RICH		NO LOUD, CROWDED, FAR PLACES		DRAGGING/ LAGGING		EDGY, DEEP, DULL, ACHY		PULSING, THROBBING, SHOOTING, STABBING, BURNING		

Date	Time	Color Scale Number	Symptom Area	Precipitating Event	Coping Strategy	Meds	Results

Weekly Pain Log

WEEK OF ____________

0 1	2 3	4 5	6 7	8 9 10
LOW THREAT	GUARDED	ELEVATED	HIGH ALERT	SEVERE
LIFE IS RICH	NO LOUD, CROWDED, FAR PLACES	DRAGGING/ LAGGING	EDGY, DEEP, DULL, ACHY	PULSING, THROBBING, SHOOTING, STABBING, BURNING

Date	Time	Color Scale Number	Symptom Area	Precipitating Event	Coping Strategy	Meds	Results

Weekly Pain Log

WEEK OF ____________

0	1	2	3	4	5	6	7	8	9	10
LOW THREAT		GUARDED		ELEVATED		HIGH ALERT		SEVERE		
LIFE IS RICH		NO LOUD, CROWDED, FAR PLACES		DRAGGING/ LAGGING		EDGY, DEEP, DULL, ACHY		PULSING, THROBBING, SHOOTING, STABBING, BURNING		

Date	Time	Color Scale Number	Symptom Area	Precipitating Event	Coping Strategy	Meds	Results

Weekly Pain Log

WEEK OF ____________________

0	1	2	3	4	5	6	7	8	9	10
LOW THREAT		GUARDED		ELEVATED		HIGH ALERT		SEVERE		
LIFE IS RICH		NO LOUD, CROWDED, FAR PLACES		DRAGGING/ LAGGING		EDGY, DEEP, DULL, ACHY		PULSING, THROBBING, SHOOTING, STABBING, BURNING		

Date	Time	Color Scale Number	Symptom Area	Precipitating Event	Coping Strategy	Meds	Results

Weekly Pain Log

WEEK OF ______________

0 1	2 3	4 5	6 7	8 9 10
LOW THREAT	GUARDED	ELEVATED	HIGH ALERT	SEVERE
LIFE IS RICH	NO LOUD, CROWDED, FAR PLACES	DRAGGING/ LAGGING	EDGY, DEEP, DULL, ACHY	PULSING, THROBBING, SHOOTING, STABBING, BURNING

Date	Time	Color Scale Number	Symptom Area	Precipitating Event	Coping Strategy	Meds	Results

Weekly Pain Log

WEEK OF ____________

0 1	2 3	4 5	6 7	8 9 10
LOW THREAT	**GUARDED**	**ELEVATED**	**HIGH ALERT**	**SEVERE**
LIFE IS RICH	NO LOUD, CROWDED, FAR PLACES	DRAGGING/ LAGGING	EDGY, DEEP, DULL, ACHY	PULSING, THROBBING, SHOOTING, STABBING, BURNING

Date	Time	Color Scale Number	Symptom Area	Precipitating Event	Coping Strategy	Meds	Results

Weekly Pain Log

WEEK OF ____________

0 1	2 3	4 5	6 7	8 9 10
LOW THREAT	GUARDED	ELEVATED	HIGH ALERT	SEVERE
LIFE IS RICH	NO LOUD, CROWDED, FAR PLACES	DRAGGING/ LAGGING	EDGY, DEEP, DULL, ACHY	PULSING, THROBBING, SHOOTING, STABBING, BURNING

Date	Time	Color Scale Number	Symptom Area	Precipitating Event	Coping Strategy	Meds	Results

Weekly Pain Log

WEEK OF ____________________

0	1	2	3	4	5	6	7	8	9	10
LOW THREAT		GUARDED		ELEVATED		HIGH ALERT		SEVERE		
LIFE IS RICH		NO LOUD, CROWDED, FAR PLACES		DRAGGING/ LAGGING		EDGY, DEEP, DULL, ACHY		PULSING, THROBBING, SHOOTING, STABBING, BURNING		

Date	Time	Color Scale Number	Symptom Area	Precipitating Event	Coping Strategy	Meds	Results

Weekly Pain Log

WEEK OF ____________

0 1	2 3	4 5	6 7	8 9 10
LOW THREAT	GUARDED	ELEVATED	HIGH ALERT	SEVERE
LIFE IS RICH	NO LOUD, CROWDED, FAR PLACES	DRAGGING/ LAGGING	EDGY, DEEP, DULL, ACHY	PULSING, THROBBING, SHOOTING, STABBING, BURNING

Date	Time	Color Scale Number	Symptom Area	Precipitating Event	Coping Strategy	Meds	Results

Weekly Pain Log

WEEK OF ______________

0 1	2 3	4 5	6 7	8 9 10
LOW THREAT	GUARDED	ELEVATED	HIGH ALERT	SEVERE
LIFE IS RICH	NO LOUD, CROWDED, FAR PLACES	DRAGGING/ LAGGING	EDGY, DEEP, DULL, ACHY	PULSING, THROBBING, SHOOTING, STABBING, BURNING

Date	Time	Color Scale Number	Symptom Area	Precipitating Event	Coping Strategy	Meds	Results

Weekly Pain Log

WEEK OF ______________

0	1	2	3	4	5	6	7	8	9	10
LOW THREAT		GUARDED		ELEVATED		HIGH ALERT		SEVERE		
LIFE IS RICH		NO LOUD, CROWDED, FAR PLACES		DRAGGING/ LAGGING		EDGY, DEEP, DULL, ACHY		PULSING, THROBBING, SHOOTING, STABBING, BURNING		

Date	Time	Color Scale Number	Symptom Area	Precipitating Event	Coping Strategy	Meds	Results

Weekly Pain Log

WEEK OF ____________

0 1	2 3	4 5	6 7	8 9 10
LOW THREAT	GUARDED	ELEVATED	HIGH ALERT	SEVERE
LIFE IS RICH	NO LOUD, CROWDED, FAR PLACES	DRAGGING/ LAGGING	EDGY, DEEP, DULL, ACHY	PULSING, THROBBING, SHOOTING, STABBING, BURNING

Date	Time	Color Scale Number	Symptom Area	Precipitating Event	Coping Strategy	Meds	Results

Weekly Pain Log

WEEK OF ____________

0	1	2	3	4	5	6	7	8	9	10
LOW THREAT		GUARDED		ELEVATED		HIGH ALERT		SEVERE		
LIFE IS RICH		NO LOUD, CROWDED, FAR PLACES		DRAGGING/ LAGGING		EDGY, DEEP, DULL, ACHY		PULSING, THROBBING, SHOOTING, STABBING, BURNING		

Date	Time	Color Scale Number	Symptom Area	Precipitating Event	Coping Strategy	Meds	Results

Weekly Pain Log

WEEK OF ____________________

0	1	2	3	4	5	6	7	8	9	10
LOW THREAT		GUARDED		ELEVATED		HIGH ALERT		SEVERE		
LIFE IS RICH		NO LOUD, CROWDED, FAR PLACES		DRAGGING/ LAGGING		EDGY, DEEP, DULL, ACHY		PULSING, THROBBING, SHOOTING, STABBING, BURNING		

Date	Time	Color Scale Number	Symptom Area	Precipitating Event	Coping Strategy	Meds	Results

Weekly Pain Log

WEEK OF ______________

0	1	2	3	4	5	6	7	8	9	10
LOW THREAT		GUARDED		ELEVATED		HIGH ALERT		SEVERE		
LIFE IS RICH		NO LOUD, CROWDED, FAR PLACES		DRAGGING/ LAGGING		EDGY, DEEP, DULL, ACHY		PULSING, THROBBING, SHOOTING, STABBING, BURNING		

Date	Time	Color Scale Number	Symptom Area	Precipitating Event	Coping Strategy	Meds	Results

Weekly Pain Log

WEEK OF ______________________

0	1	2	3	4	5	6	7	8	9	10
LOW THREAT		GUARDED		ELEVATED		HIGH ALERT		SEVERE		
LIFE IS RICH		NO LOUD, CROWDED, FAR PLACES		DRAGGING/ LAGGING		EDGY, DEEP, DULL, ACHY		PULSING, THROBBING, SHOOTING, STABBING, BURNING		

Date	Time	Color Scale Number	Symptom Area	Precipitating Event	Coping Strategy	Meds	Results

Weekly Pain Log

VEEK OF ____________

0	1	2	3	4	5	6	7	8	9	10

LOW THREAT	GUARDED	ELEVATED	HIGH ALERT	SEVERE
LIFE IS RICH	NO LOUD, CROWDED, FAR PLACES	DRAGGING/ LAGGING	EDGY, DEEP, DULL, ACHY	PULSING, THROBBING, SHOOTING, STABBING, BURNING

Date	Time	Color Scale Number	Symptom Area	Precipitating Event	Coping Strategy	Meds	Results

Weekly Pain Log

WEEK OF ____________

0 1	2 3	4 5	6 7	8 9 10
LOW THREAT	GUARDED	ELEVATED	HIGH ALERT	SEVERE
LIFE IS RICH	NO LOUD, CROWDED, FAR PLACES	DRAGGING/ LAGGING	EDGY, DEEP, DULL, ACHY	PULSING, THROBBING, SHOOTING, STABBING, BURNING

Date	Time	Color Scale Number	Symptom Area	Precipitating Event	Coping Strategy	Meds	Results

Weekly Pain Log

WEEK OF ____________

0	1	2	3	4	5	6	7	8	9	10
LOW THREAT		GUARDED		ELEVATED		HIGH ALERT		SEVERE		
LIFE IS RICH		NO LOUD, CROWDED, FAR PLACES		DRAGGING/ LAGGING		EDGY, DEEP, DULL, ACHY		PULSING, THROBBING, SHOOTING, STABBING, BURNING		

Date	Time	Color Scale Number	Symptom Area	Precipitating Event	Coping Strategy	Meds	Results

Weekly Pain Log

WEEK OF ______________________

0 1	2 3	4 5	6 7	8 9 10
LOW THREAT	**GUARDED**	**ELEVATED**	**HIGH ALERT**	**SEVERE**
LIFE IS RICH	NO LOUD, CROWDED, FAR PLACES	DRAGGING/ LAGGING	EDGY, DEEP, DULL, ACHY	PULSING, THROBBING, SHOOTING, STABBING, BURNING

Date	Time	Color Scale Number	Symptom Area	Precipitating Event	Coping Strategy	Meds	Results

Weekly Pain Log

WEEK OF ____________________

0 1	2 3	4 5	6 7	8 9 10
LOW THREAT	GUARDED	ELEVATED	HIGH ALERT	SEVERE
LIFE IS RICH	NO LOUD, CROWDED, FAR PLACES	DRAGGING/ LAGGING	EDGY, DEEP, DULL, ACHY	PULSING, THROBBING, SHOOTING, STABBING, BURNING

Date	Time	Color Scale Number	Symptom Area	Precipitating Event	Coping Strategy	Meds	Results

Weekly Pain Log

WEEK OF ____________________

0	1	2	3	4	5	6	7	8	9	10
LOW THREAT		GUARDED		ELEVATED		HIGH ALERT		SEVERE		
LIFE IS RICH		NO LOUD, CROWDED, FAR PLACES		DRAGGING/ LAGGING		EDGY, DEEP, DULL, ACHY		PULSING, THROBBING, SHOOTING, STABBING, BURNING		

Date	Time	Color Scale Number	Symptom Area	Precipitating Event	Coping Strategy	Meds	Results

Weekly Pain Log

WEEK OF ____________

0 1	2 3	4 5	6 7	8 9 10
LOW THREAT	GUARDED	ELEVATED	HIGH ALERT	SEVERE
LIFE IS RICH	NO LOUD, CROWDED, FAR PLACES	DRAGGING/ LAGGING	EDGY, DEEP, DULL, ACHY	PULSING, THROBBING, SHOOTING, STABBING, BURNING

Date	Time	Color Scale Number	Symptom Area	Precipitating Event	Coping Strategy	Meds	Results

Weekly Pain Log

WEEK OF ____________________

0	1	2	3	4	5	6	7	8	9	10

LOW THREAT	GUARDED	ELEVATED	HIGH ALERT	SEVERE
LIFE IS RICH	NO LOUD, CROWDED, FAR PLACES	DRAGGING/ LAGGING	EDGY, DEEP, DULL, ACHY	PULSING, THROBBING, SHOOTING, STABBING, BURNING

Date	Time	Color Scale Number	Symptom Area	Precipitating Event	Coping Strategy	Meds	Results

Weekly Pain Log

WEEK OF ______________

0 1	2 3	4 5	6 7	8 9 10
LOW THREAT	GUARDED	ELEVATED	HIGH ALERT	SEVERE
LIFE IS RICH	NO LOUD, CROWDED, FAR PLACES	DRAGGING/ LAGGING	EDGY, DEEP, DULL, ACHY	PULSING, THROBBING, SHOOTING, STABBING, BURNING

Date	Time	Color Scale Number	Symptom Area	Precipitating Event	Coping Strategy	Meds	Results

Weekly Pain Log

WEEK OF ____________________

0 – 1	2 – 3	4 – 5	6 – 7	8 – 9 – 10
LOW THREAT	GUARDED	ELEVATED	HIGH ALERT	SEVERE
LIFE IS RICH	NO LOUD, CROWDED, FAR PLACES	DRAGGING/ LAGGING	EDGY, DEEP, DULL, ACHY	PULSING, THROBBING, SHOOTING, STABBING, BURNING

Date	Time	Color Scale Number	Symptom Area	Precipitating Event	Coping Strategy	Meds	Results

Weekly Pain Log

WEEK OF ____________

0	1	2	3	4	5	6	7	8	9	10
LOW THREAT		GUARDED		ELEVATED		HIGH ALERT		SEVERE		
LIFE IS RICH		NO LOUD, CROWDED, FAR PLACES		DRAGGING/ LAGGING		EDGY, DEEP, DULL, ACHY		PULSING, THROBBING, SHOOTING, STABBING, BURNING		

Date	Time	Color Scale Number	Symptom Area	Precipitating Event	Coping Strategy	Meds	Results

Weekly Pain Log

WEEK OF ____________

0	1	2	3	4	5	6	7	8	9	10
LOW THREAT		GUARDED		ELEVATED		HIGH ALERT		SEVERE		
LIFE IS RICH		NO LOUD, CROWDED, FAR PLACES		DRAGGING/ LAGGING		EDGY, DEEP, DULL, ACHY		PULSING, THROBBING, SHOOTING, STABBING, BURNING		

Date	Time	Color Scale Number	Symptom Area	Precipitating Event	Coping Strategy	Meds	Results

Weekly Pain Log

WEEK OF ______________

0 1	2 3	4 5	6 7	8 9 10
LOW THREAT	GUARDED	ELEVATED	HIGH ALERT	SEVERE
LIFE IS RICH	NO LOUD, CROWDED, FAR PLACES	DRAGGING/ LAGGING	EDGY, DEEP, DULL, ACHY	PULSING, THROBBING, SHOOTING, STABBING, BURNING

Date	Time	Color Scale Number	Symptom Area	Precipitating Event	Coping Strategy	Meds	Results

Weekly Pain Log

WEEK OF ________________

0	1	2	3	4	5	6	7	8	9	10
LOW THREAT		GUARDED		ELEVATED		HIGH ALERT		SEVERE		
LIFE IS RICH		NO LOUD, CROWDED, FAR PLACES		DRAGGING/ LAGGING		EDGY, DEEP, DULL, ACHY		PULSING, THROBBING, SHOOTING, STABBING, BURNING		

Date	Time	Color Scale Number	Symptom Area	Precipitating Event	Coping Strategy	Meds	Results

Weekly Pain Log

WEEK OF ______________

0	1	2	3	4	5	6	7	8	9	10
LOW THREAT		GUARDED		ELEVATED		HIGH ALERT		SEVERE		
LIFE IS RICH		NO LOUD, CROWDED, FAR PLACES		DRAGGING/ LAGGING		EDGY, DEEP, DULL, ACHY		PULSING, THROBBING, SHOOTING, STABBING, BURNING		

Date	Time	Color Scale Number	Symptom Area	Precipitating Event	Coping Strategy	Meds	Results

Weekly Pain Log

WEEK OF ______________

0 1	2 3	4 5	6 7	8 9 10
LOW THREAT	GUARDED	ELEVATED	HIGH ALERT	SEVERE
LIFE IS RICH	NO LOUD, CROWDED, FAR PLACES	DRAGGING/ LAGGING	EDGY, DEEP, DULL, ACHY	PULSING, THROBBING, SHOOTING, STABBING, BURNING

Date	Time	Color Scale Number	Symptom Area	Precipitating Event	Coping Strategy	Meds	Results

Weekly Pain Log

WEEK OF ____________

0 1	2 3	4 5	6 7	8 9 10
LOW THREAT	GUARDED	ELEVATED	HIGH ALERT	SEVERE
LIFE IS RICH	NO LOUD, CROWDED, FAR PLACES	DRAGGING/ LAGGING	EDGY, DEEP, DULL, ACHY	PULSING, THROBBING, SHOOTING, STABBING, BURNING

Date	Time	Color Scale Number	Symptom Area	Precipitating Event	Coping Strategy	Meds	Results

Weekly Pain Log

WEEK OF ______________________

0 1	2 3	4 5	6 7	8 9 10
LOW THREAT	GUARDED	ELEVATED	HIGH ALERT	SEVERE
LIFE IS RICH	NO LOUD, CROWDED, FAR PLACES	DRAGGING/ LAGGING	EDGY, DEEP, DULL, ACHY	PULSING, THROBBING, SHOOTING, STABBING, BURNING

Date	Time	Color Scale Number	Symptom Area	Precipitating Event	Coping Strategy	Meds	Results

Weekly Pain Log

WEEK OF ____________

0	1	2	3	4	5	6	7	8	9	10
LOW THREAT		GUARDED		ELEVATED		HIGH ALERT		SEVERE		
LIFE IS RICH		NO LOUD, CROWDED, FAR PLACES		DRAGGING/ LAGGING		EDGY, DEEP, DULL, ACHY		PULSING, THROBBING, SHOOTING, STABBING, BURNING		

Date	Time	Color Scale Number	Symptom Area	Precipitating Event	Coping Strategy	Meds	Results

Weekly Pain Log

WEEK OF ____________________

0 1	2 3	4 5	6 7	8 9 10
LOW THREAT	GUARDED	ELEVATED	HIGH ALERT	SEVERE
LIFE IS RICH	NO LOUD, CROWDED, FAR PLACES	DRAGGING/ LAGGING	EDGY, DEEP, DULL, ACHY	PULSING, THROBBING, SHOOTING, STABBING, BURNING

Date	Time	Color Scale Number	Symptom Area	Precipitating Event	Coping Strategy	Meds	Results

Weekly Pain Log

VEEK OF ____________

0	1	2	3	4	5	6	7	8	9	10
LOW THREAT		GUARDED		ELEVATED		HIGH ALERT		SEVERE		
LIFE IS RICH		NO LOUD, CROWDED, FAR PLACES		DRAGGING/ LAGGING		EDGY, DEEP, DULL, ACHY		PULSING, THROBBING, SHOOTING, STABBING, BURNING		

Date	Time	Color Scale Number	Symptom Area	Precipitating Event	Coping Strategy	Meds	Results

Weekly Pain Log

WEEK OF ____________________

0 1	2 3	4 5	6 7	8 9 10
LOW THREAT	**GUARDED**	**ELEVATED**	**HIGH ALERT**	**SEVERE**
LIFE IS RICH	NO LOUD, CROWDED, FAR PLACES	DRAGGING/ LAGGING	EDGY, DEEP, DULL, ACHY	PULSING, THROBBING, SHOOTING, STABBING, BURNING

Date	Time	Color Scale Number	Symptom Area	Precipitating Event	Coping Strategy	Meds	Results

Weekly Pain Log

WEEK OF ____________

0 1	2 3	4 5	6 7	8 9 10
LOW THREAT	GUARDED	ELEVATED	HIGH ALERT	SEVERE
LIFE IS RICH	NO LOUD, CROWDED, FAR PLACES	DRAGGING/ LAGGING	EDGY, DEEP, DULL, ACHY	PULSING, THROBBING, SHOOTING, STABBING, BURNING

Date	Time	Color Scale Number	Symptom Area	Precipitating Event	Coping Strategy	Meds	Results

Weekly Pain Log

WEEK OF ____________________

0	1	2	3	4	5	6	7	8	9	10
LOW THREAT		GUARDED		ELEVATED		HIGH ALERT		SEVERE		
LIFE IS RICH		NO LOUD, CROWDED, FAR PLACES		DRAGGING/ LAGGING		EDGY, DEEP, DULL, ACHY		PULSING, THROBBING, SHOOTING, STABBING, BURNING		

Date	Time	Color Scale Number	Symptom Area	Precipitating Event	Coping Strategy	Meds	Results

Weekly Pain Log

WEEK OF ______________

0	1	2	3	4	5	6	7	8	9	10
LOW THREAT		GUARDED		ELEVATED		HIGH ALERT		SEVERE		
LIFE IS RICH		NO LOUD, CROWDED, FAR PLACES		DRAGGING/ LAGGING		EDGY, DEEP, DULL, ACHY		PULSING, THROBBING, SHOOTING, STABBING, BURNING		

Date	Time	Color Scale Number	Symptom Area	Precipitating Event	Coping Strategy	Meds	Results

Weekly Pain Log

WEEK OF ____________________

0	1	2	3	4	5	6	7	8	9	10
LOW THREAT		GUARDED		ELEVATED		HIGH ALERT		SEVERE		
LIFE IS RICH		NO LOUD, CROWDED, FAR PLACES		DRAGGING/ LAGGING		EDGY, DEEP, DULL, ACHY		PULSING, THROBBING, SHOOTING, STABBING, BURNING		

Date	Time	Color Scale Number	Symptom Area	Precipitating Event	Coping Strategy	Meds	Results

Weekly Pain Log

WEEK OF ____________

0 1	2 3	4 5	6 7	8 9 10
LOW THREAT	GUARDED	ELEVATED	HIGH ALERT	SEVERE
LIFE IS RICH	NO LOUD, CROWDED, FAR PLACES	DRAGGING/ LAGGING	EDGY, DEEP, DULL, ACHY	PULSING, THROBBING, SHOOTING, STABBING, BURNING

Date	Time	Color Scale Number	Symptom Area	Precipitating Event	Coping Strategy	Meds	Results

Weekly Pain Log

WEEK OF ____________________

0 1	2 3	4 5	6 7	8 9 10
LOW THREAT	GUARDED	ELEVATED	HIGH ALERT	SEVERE
LIFE IS RICH	NO LOUD, CROWDED, FAR PLACES	DRAGGING/ LAGGING	EDGY, DEEP, DULL, ACHY	PULSING, THROBBING, SHOOTING, STABBING, BURNING

Date	Time	Color Scale Number	Symptom Area	Precipitating Event	Coping Strategy	Meds	Results

Weekly Pain Log

WEEK OF ______________

0	1	2	3	4	5	6	7	8	9	10
LOW THREAT		GUARDED		ELEVATED		HIGH ALERT		SEVERE		
LIFE IS RICH		NO LOUD, CROWDED, FAR PLACES		DRAGGING/ LAGGING		EDGY, DEEP, DULL, ACHY		PULSING, THROBBING, SHOOTING, STABBING, BURNING		

Date	Time	Color Scale Number	Symptom Area	Precipitating Event	Coping Strategy	Meds	Results

Weekly Pain Log

WEEK OF ____________

0	1	2	3	4	5	6	7	8	9	10
LOW THREAT		GUARDED		ELEVATED		HIGH ALERT		SEVERE		
LIFE IS RICH		NO LOUD, CROWDED, FAR PLACES		DRAGGING/ LAGGING		EDGY, DEEP, DULL, ACHY		PULSING, THROBBING, SHOOTING, STABBING, BURNING		

Date	Time	Color Scale Number	Symptom Area	Precipitating Event	Coping Strategy	Meds	Results

Weekly Pain Log

WEEK OF ______________

0	1	2	3	4	5	6	7	8	9	10
LOW THREAT		GUARDED		ELEVATED		HIGH ALERT		SEVERE		
LIFE IS RICH		NO LOUD, CROWDED, FAR PLACES		DRAGGING/ LAGGING		EDGY, DEEP, DULL, ACHY		PULSING, THROBBING, SHOOTING, STABBING, BURNING		

Date	Time	Color Scale Number	Symptom Area	Precipitating Event	Coping Strategy	Meds	Results

Weekly Pain Log

WEEK OF ____________________

0 1	2 3	4 5	6 7	8 9 10
LOW THREAT	GUARDED	ELEVATED	HIGH ALERT	SEVERE
LIFE IS RICH	NO LOUD, CROWDED, FAR PLACES	DRAGGING/ LAGGING	EDGY, DEEP, DULL, ACHY	PULSING, THROBBING, SHOOTING, STABBING, BURNING

Date	Time	Color Scale Number	Symptom Area	Precipitating Event	Coping Strategy	Meds	Results

Weekly Pain Log

WEEK OF ____________

0	1	2	3	4	5	6	7	8	9	10
LOW THREAT		GUARDED		ELEVATED		HIGH ALERT		SEVERE		
LIFE IS RICH		NO LOUD, CROWDED, FAR PLACES		DRAGGING/ LAGGING		EDGY, DEEP, DULL, ACHY		PULSING, THROBBING, SHOOTING, STABBING, BURNING		

Date	Time	Color Scale Number	Symptom Area	Precipitating Event	Coping Strategy	Meds	Results

Weekly Pain Log

WEEK OF ______________________

0 1	2 3	4 5	6 7	8 9 10
LOW THREAT	GUARDED	ELEVATED	HIGH ALERT	SEVERE
LIFE IS RICH	NO LOUD, CROWDED, FAR PLACES	DRAGGING/ LAGGING	EDGY, DEEP, DULL, ACHY	PULSING, THROBBING, SHOOTING, STABBING, BURNING

Date	Time	Color Scale Number	Symptom Area	Precipitating Event	Coping Strategy	Meds	Results

Weekly Pain Log

WEEK OF ____________

0	1	2	3	4	5	6	7	8	9	10

LOW THREAT	GUARDED	ELEVATED	HIGH ALERT	SEVERE
LIFE IS RICH	NO LOUD, CROWDED, FAR PLACES	DRAGGING/ LAGGING	EDGY, DEEP, DULL, ACHY	PULSING, THROBBING, SHOOTING, STABBING, BURNING

Date	Time	Color Scale Number	Symptom Area	Precipitating Event	Coping Strategy	Meds	Results

Weekly Pain Log

WEEK OF ____________________

0	1	2	3	4	5	6	7	8	9	10
LOW THREAT		GUARDED		ELEVATED		HIGH ALERT		SEVERE		
LIFE IS RICH		NO LOUD, CROWDED, FAR PLACES		DRAGGING/ LAGGING		EDGY, DEEP, DULL, ACHY		PULSING, THROBBING, SHOOTING, STABBING, BURNING		

Date	Time	Color Scale Number	Symptom Area	Precipitating Event	Coping Strategy	Meds	Results

Weekly Pain Log

WEEK OF ____________

0	1	2	3	4	5	6	7	8	9	10
LOW THREAT		GUARDED		ELEVATED		HIGH ALERT		SEVERE		
LIFE IS RICH		NO LOUD, CROWDED, FAR PLACES		DRAGGING/ LAGGING		EDGY, DEEP, DULL, ACHY		PULSING, THROBBING, SHOOTING, STABBING, BURNING		

Date	Time	Color Scale Number	Symptom Area	Precipitating Event	Coping Strategy	Meds	Results

Weekly Pain Log

WEEK OF ____________________

0	1	2	3	4	5	6	7	8	9	10
LOW THREAT		GUARDED		ELEVATED		HIGH ALERT		SEVERE		
LIFE IS RICH		NO LOUD, CROWDED, FAR PLACES		DRAGGING/ LAGGING		EDGY, DEEP, DULL, ACHY		PULSING, THROBBING, SHOOTING, STABBING, BURNING		

Date	Time	Color Scale Number	Symptom Area	Precipitating Event	Coping Strategy	Meds	Results

Weekly Pain Log

WEEK OF ____________

0	1	2	3	4	5	6	7	8	9	10
LOW THREAT		GUARDED		ELEVATED		HIGH ALERT		SEVERE		
LIFE IS RICH		NO LOUD, CROWDED, FAR PLACES		DRAGGING/ LAGGING		EDGY, DEEP, DULL, ACHY		PULSING, THROBBING, SHOOTING, STABBING, BURNING		

Date	Time	Color Scale Number	Symptom Area	Precipitating Event	Coping Strategy	Meds	Results

Weekly Pain Log

WEEK OF ____________________

0	1	2	3	4	5	6	7	8	9	10
LOW THREAT		GUARDED		ELEVATED		HIGH ALERT		SEVERE		
LIFE IS RICH		NO LOUD, CROWDED, FAR PLACES		DRAGGING/ LAGGING		EDGY, DEEP, DULL, ACHY		PULSING, THROBBING, SHOOTING, STABBING, BURNING		

Date	Time	Color Scale Number	Symptom Area	Precipitating Event	Coping Strategy	Meds	Results

Weekly Pain Log

WEEK OF ____________

0	1	2	3	4	5	6	7	8	9	10
LOW THREAT		GUARDED		ELEVATED		HIGH ALERT		SEVERE		
LIFE IS RICH		NO LOUD, CROWDED, FAR PLACES		DRAGGING/ LAGGING		EDGY, DEEP, DULL, ACHY		PULSING, THROBBING, SHOOTING, STABBING, BURNING		

Date	Time	Color Scale Number	Symptom Area	Precipitating Event	Coping Strategy	Meds	Results

Weekly Pain Log

WEEK OF ____________________

0 1	2 3	4 5	6 7	8 9 10
LOW THREAT	GUARDED	ELEVATED	HIGH ALERT	SEVERE
LIFE IS RICH	NO LOUD, CROWDED, FAR PLACES	DRAGGING/ LAGGING	EDGY, DEEP, DULL, ACHY	PULSING, THROBBING, SHOOTING, STABBING, BURNING

Date	Time	Color Scale Number	Symptom Area	Precipitating Event	Coping Strategy	Meds	Results

Weekly Pain Log

WEEK OF ____________

0 1	2 3	4 5	6 7	8 9 10
LOW THREAT	GUARDED	ELEVATED	HIGH ALERT	SEVERE
LIFE IS RICH	NO LOUD, CROWDED, FAR PLACES	DRAGGING/ LAGGING	EDGY, DEEP, DULL, ACHY	PULSING, THROBBING, SHOOTING, STABBING, BURNING

Date	Time	Color Scale Number	Symptom Area	Precipitating Event	Coping Strategy	Meds	Results

Weekly Pain Log

WEEK OF ______________

0	1	2	3	4	5	6	7	8	9	10
LOW THREAT		GUARDED		ELEVATED		HIGH ALERT		SEVERE		
LIFE IS RICH		NO LOUD, CROWDED, FAR PLACES		DRAGGING/ LAGGING		EDGY, DEEP, DULL, ACHY		PULSING, THROBBING, SHOOTING, STABBING, BURNING		

Date	Time	Color Scale Number	Symptom Area	Precipitating Event	Coping Strategy	Meds	Results

Weekly Pain Log

WEEK OF ______________

0	1	2	3	4	5	6	7	8	9	10
LOW THREAT		GUARDED		ELEVATED		HIGH ALERT		SEVERE		
LIFE IS RICH		NO LOUD, CROWDED, FAR PLACES		DRAGGING/ LAGGING		EDGY, DEEP, DULL, ACHY		PULSING, THROBBING, SHOOTING, STABBING, BURNING		

Date	Time	Color Scale Number	Symptom Area	Precipitating Event	Coping Strategy	Meds	Results

Weekly Pain Log

WEEK OF ____________________

0	1	2	3	4	5	6	7	8	9	10
LOW THREAT		GUARDED		ELEVATED		HIGH ALERT		SEVERE		
LIFE IS RICH		NO LOUD, CROWDED, FAR PLACES		DRAGGING/ LAGGING		EDGY, DEEP, DULL, ACHY		PULSING, THROBBING, SHOOTING, STABBING, BURNING		

Date	Time	Color Scale Number	Symptom Area	Precipitating Event	Coping Strategy	Meds	Results

Weekly Pain Log

WEEK OF ____________

0	1	2	3	4	5	6	7	8	9	10
LOW THREAT		GUARDED		ELEVATED		HIGH ALERT		SEVERE		
LIFE IS RICH		NO LOUD, CROWDED, FAR PLACES		DRAGGING/ LAGGING		EDGY, DEEP, DULL, ACHY		PULSING, THROBBING, SHOOTING, STABBING, BURNING		

Date	Time	Color Scale Number	Symptom Area	Precipitating Event	Coping Strategy	Meds	Results

Weekly Pain Log

WEEK OF ____________________

0	1	2	3	4	5	6	7	8	9	10
LOW THREAT		GUARDED		ELEVATED		HIGH ALERT		SEVERE		
LIFE IS RICH		NO LOUD, CROWDED, FAR PLACES		DRAGGING/ LAGGING		EDGY, DEEP, DULL, ACHY		PULSING, THROBBING, SHOOTING, STABBING, BURNING		

Date	Time	Color Scale Number	Symptom Area	Precipitating Event	Coping Strategy	Meds	Results

Weekly Pain Log

WEEK OF ______________

0	1	2	3	4	5	6	7	8	9	10
LOW THREAT		GUARDED		ELEVATED		HIGH ALERT		SEVERE		
LIFE IS RICH		NO LOUD, CROWDED, FAR PLACES		DRAGGING/ LAGGING		EDGY, DEEP, DULL, ACHY		PULSING, THROBBING, SHOOTING, STABBING, BURNING		

Date	Time	Color Scale Number	Symptom Area	Precipitating Event	Coping Strategy	Meds	Results

Weekly Pain Log

WEEK OF ____________________

0 1	2 3	4 5	6 7	8 9 10
LOW THREAT	GUARDED	ELEVATED	HIGH ALERT	SEVERE
LIFE IS RICH	NO LOUD, CROWDED, FAR PLACES	DRAGGING/ LAGGING	EDGY, DEEP, DULL, ACHY	PULSING, THROBBING, SHOOTING, STABBING, BURNING

Date	Time	Color Scale Number	Symptom Area	Precipitating Event	Coping Strategy	Meds	Results

Weekly Pain Log

WEEK OF ______________

0	1	2	3	4	5	6	7	8	9	10

LOW THREAT	GUARDED	ELEVATED	HIGH ALERT	SEVERE
LIFE IS RICH	NO LOUD, CROWDED, FAR PLACES	DRAGGING/ LAGGING	EDGY, DEEP, DULL, ACHY	PULSING, THROBBING, SHOOTING, STABBING, BURNING

Date	Time	Color Scale Number	Symptom Area	Precipitating Event	Coping Strategy	Meds	Results

Weekly Pain Log

WEEK OF ____________

0 1	2 3	4 5	6 7	8 9 10
LOW THREAT	GUARDED	ELEVATED	HIGH ALERT	SEVERE
LIFE IS RICH	NO LOUD, CROWDED, FAR PLACES	DRAGGING/ LAGGING	EDGY, DEEP, DULL, ACHY	PULSING, THROBBING, SHOOTING, STABBING, BURNING

Date	Time	Color Scale Number	Symptom Area	Precipitating Event	Coping Strategy	Meds	Results

Weekly Pain Log

WEEK OF ______________

0	1	2	3	4	5	6	7	8	9	10
LOW THREAT		GUARDED		ELEVATED		HIGH ALERT		SEVERE		
LIFE IS RICH		NO LOUD, CROWDED, FAR PLACES		DRAGGING/ LAGGING		EDGY, DEEP, DULL, ACHY		PULSING, THROBBING, SHOOTING, STABBING, BURNING		

Date	Time	Color Scale Number	Symptom Area	Precipitating Event	Coping Strategy	Meds	Results

Weekly Pain Log

WEEK OF ____________

0	1	2	3	4	5	6	7	8	9	10

LOW THREAT	GUARDED	ELEVATED	HIGH ALERT	SEVERE
LIFE IS RICH	NO LOUD, CROWDED, FAR PLACES	DRAGGING/ LAGGING	EDGY, DEEP, DULL, ACHY	PULSING, THROBBING, SHOOTING, STABBING, BURNING

Date	Time	Color Scale Number	Symptom Area	Precipitating Event	Coping Strategy	Meds	Results

Weekly Pain Log

WEEK OF ____________

0	1	2	3	4	5	6	7	8	9	10
LOW THREAT		GUARDED		ELEVATED		HIGH ALERT		SEVERE		
LIFE IS RICH		NO LOUD, CROWDED, FAR PLACES		DRAGGING/ LAGGING		EDGY, DEEP, DULL, ACHY		PULSING, THROBBING, SHOOTING, STABBING, BURNING		

Date	Time	Color Scale Number	Symptom Area	Precipitating Event	Coping Strategy	Meds	Results

Weekly Pain Log

WEEK OF ______________________

0 1	2 3	4 5	6 7	8 9 10
LOW THREAT	GUARDED	ELEVATED	HIGH ALERT	SEVERE
LIFE IS RICH	NO LOUD, CROWDED, FAR PLACES	DRAGGING/ LAGGING	EDGY, DEEP, DULL, ACHY	PULSING, THROBBING, SHOOTING, STABBING, BURNING

Date	Time	Color Scale Number	Symptom Area	Precipitating Event	Coping Strategy	Meds	Results

Weekly Pain Log

WEEK OF ______________

0 1	2 3	4 5	6 7	8 9 10
LOW THREAT	GUARDED	ELEVATED	HIGH ALERT	SEVERE
LIFE IS RICH	NO LOUD, CROWDED, FAR PLACES	DRAGGING/ LAGGING	EDGY, DEEP, DULL, ACHY	PULSING, THROBBING, SHOOTING, STABBING, BURNING

Date	Time	Color Scale Number	Symptom Area	Precipitating Event	Coping Strategy	Meds	Results

Weekly Pain Log

WEEK OF ____________________

0 – 1	2 – 3	4 – 5	6 – 7	8 – 9 – 10
LOW THREAT	GUARDED	ELEVATED	HIGH ALERT	SEVERE
LIFE IS RICH	NO LOUD, CROWDED, FAR PLACES	DRAGGING/ LAGGING	EDGY, DEEP, DULL, ACHY	PULSING, THROBBING, SHOOTING, STABBING, BURNING

Date	Time	Color Scale Number	Symptom Area	Precipitating Event	Coping Strategy	Meds	Results

Weekly Pain Log

WEEK OF ____________

0 1	2 3	4 5	6 7	8 9 10
LOW THREAT	GUARDED	ELEVATED	HIGH ALERT	SEVERE
LIFE IS RICH	NO LOUD, CROWDED, FAR PLACES	DRAGGING/ LAGGING	EDGY, DEEP, DULL, ACHY	PULSING, THROBBING, SHOOTING, STABBING, BURNING

Date	Time	Color Scale Number	Symptom Area	Precipitating Event	Coping Strategy	Meds	Results

Weekly Pain Log

WEEK OF ______________________

0 1	2 3	4 5	6 7	8 9 10
LOW THREAT	GUARDED	ELEVATED	HIGH ALERT	SEVERE
LIFE IS RICH	NO LOUD, CROWDED, FAR PLACES	DRAGGING/ LAGGING	EDGY, DEEP, DULL, ACHY	PULSING, THROBBING, SHOOTING, STABBING, BURNING

Date	Time	Color Scale Number	Symptom Area	Precipitating Event	Coping Strategy	Meds	Results

Weekly Pain Log

WEEK OF ____________

0 1	2 3	4 5	6 7	8 9 10
LOW THREAT	GUARDED	ELEVATED	HIGH ALERT	SEVERE
LIFE IS RICH	NO LOUD, CROWDED, FAR PLACES	DRAGGING/ LAGGING	EDGY, DEEP, DULL, ACHY	PULSING, THROBBING, SHOOTING, STABBING, BURNING

Date	Time	Color Scale Number	Symptom Area	Precipitating Event	Coping Strategy	Meds	Results

Weekly Pain Log

WEEK OF ____________________

0 1	2 3	4 5	6 7	8 9 10
LOW THREAT	GUARDED	ELEVATED	HIGH ALERT	SEVERE
LIFE IS RICH	NO LOUD, CROWDED, FAR PLACES	DRAGGING/ LAGGING	EDGY, DEEP, DULL, ACHY	PULSING, THROBBING, SHOOTING, STABBING, BURNING

Date	Time	Color Scale Number	Symptom Area	Precipitating Event	Coping Strategy	Meds	Results

Weekly Pain Log

WEEK OF ____________

0	1	2	3	4	5	6	7	8	9	10
LOW THREAT		GUARDED		ELEVATED		HIGH ALERT		SEVERE		
LIFE IS RICH		NO LOUD, CROWDED, FAR PLACES		DRAGGING/ LAGGING		EDGY, DEEP, DULL, ACHY		PULSING, THROBBING, SHOOTING, STABBING, BURNING		

Date	Time	Color Scale Number	Symptom Area	Precipitating Event	Coping Strategy	Meds	Results

Weekly Pain Log

WEEK OF ____________________

0	1	2	3	4	5	6	7	8	9	10
LOW THREAT		GUARDED		ELEVATED		HIGH ALERT		SEVERE		
LIFE IS RICH		NO LOUD, CROWDED, FAR PLACES		DRAGGING/ LAGGING		EDGY, DEEP, DULL, ACHY		PULSING, THROBBING, SHOOTING, STABBING, BURNING		

Date	Time	Color Scale Number	Symptom Area	Precipitating Event	Coping Strategy	Meds	Results

Weekly Pain Log

WEEK OF ____________

0 1	2 3	4 5	6 7	8 9 10
LOW THREAT	GUARDED	ELEVATED	HIGH ALERT	SEVERE
LIFE IS RICH	NO LOUD, CROWDED, FAR PLACES	DRAGGING/ LAGGING	EDGY, DEEP, DULL, ACHY	PULSING, THROBBING, SHOOTING, STABBING, BURNING

Date	Time	Color Scale Number	Symptom Area	Precipitating Event	Coping Strategy	Meds	Results

Weekly Pain Log

WEEK OF ____________________

0	1	2	3	4	5	6	7	8	9	10
LOW THREAT		GUARDED		ELEVATED		HIGH ALERT		SEVERE		
LIFE IS RICH		NO LOUD, CROWDED, FAR PLACES		DRAGGING/ LAGGING		EDGY, DEEP, DULL, ACHY		PULSING, THROBBING, SHOOTING, STABBING, BURNING		

Date	Time	Color Scale Number	Symptom Area	Precipitating Event	Coping Strategy	Meds	Results

Weekly Pain Log

WEEK OF ____________

0 1	2 3	4 5	6 7	8 9 10
LOW THREAT	GUARDED	ELEVATED	HIGH ALERT	SEVERE
LIFE IS RICH	NO LOUD, CROWDED, FAR PLACES	DRAGGING/ LAGGING	EDGY, DEEP, DULL, ACHY	PULSING, THROBBING, SHOOTING, STABBING, BURNING

Date	Time	Color Scale Number	Symptom Area	Precipitating Event	Coping Strategy	Meds	Results

Weekly Pain Log

WEEK OF ______________________

0	1	2	3	4	5	6	7	8	9	10
LOW THREAT		GUARDED		ELEVATED		HIGH ALERT		SEVERE		
LIFE IS RICH		NO LOUD, CROWDED, FAR PLACES		DRAGGING/ LAGGING		EDGY, DEEP, DULL, ACHY		PULSING, THROBBING, SHOOTING, STABBING, BURNING		

Date	Time	Color Scale Number	Symptom Area	Precipitating Event	Coping Strategy	Meds	Results

Made in the USA
Las Vegas, NV
07 November 2026

57673304R00074

Weekly Pain Log

WEEK OF ____________

0	1	2	3	4	5	6	7	8	9	10
LOW THREAT		GUARDED		ELEVATED		HIGH ALERT		SEVERE		
LIFE IS RICH		NO LOUD, CROWDED, FAR PLACES		DRAGGING/ LAGGING		EDGY, DEEP, DULL, ACHY		PULSING, THROBBING, SHOOTING, STABBING, BURNING		

Date	Time	Color Scale Number	Symptom Area	Precipitating Event	Coping Strategy	Meds	Results

Rich Health Solutions

www.richhealth.net

ISBN 9780997528831
90000
9 780997 528831